Essential Oils for Pain & Inflammation

Essential Oil Recipes for
Pain and Inflammation
for Diffusers, Roller Bottles,
Inhalers & more.

Rica V. Gadi

This book is dedicated to all the strong people who are taking responsibility of your own well being and doing something to be better.

All my heartfelt gratitude to the following people: my mom Ruby Jane, you have made me everything I am today; my dad Nestor-- my eternal, my angel, and the source of my perseverance; Mommyling, my spiritual guide ; Ria & Joe, the true witnesses of my transformation and my foundation pillars; Ellie Jane, the sparkle of our eyes;

Juan, thanks for always encouraging me to push harder - you are my ONE; Rocco & Radha, my reason for everything.

The Love of my family and friends is the fountain of inspiration that never runs dry. Thank you for constantly inspiring me, motivating me, and loving me unconditionally.

This book will never be complete without the help of my trusted and talented friends the #NOWsuperstars and my #oilbularya friends

Blending Essential Oils to use for a very specific reason has become very popular in the recent years. There are several reasons why this is so. Blending EOs is basically about inhaling - as it has been proven that aromas have the ability to trigger feelings, emotions and personal memories.

With this in mind, it is obvious that everyone is unique when it comes to what triggers your senses. It all boils down to personal preference for the aroma to trigger what you want to unleash. Everyone is different and we all connect to the aroma differently, so what might work for one might not work for another person.

Of course, we also want the blend we personalize to be therapeutic. This is the best reason why to blend essential oils. We want the blend we create to help us with a very specific emotion or physical condition. As much as smelling good is important in a blend, it is more important that we blend oils that is not only pleasing to the smell but also produces the therapeutic effect we are after.

Then you have to think about contraindications. Making sure the blend you create is safe to use.

I suggest that before blending find out if the oils you are using is safe for a condition you may have example, if you are pregnant, or have specific allergies. Consult your physician prior to moving forward.

The recipes I have in this book is a compilation of what has proven to work and favored by hundreds of EO enthusiasts. It takes out the guesswork to get you started.

Again, we urge you to read the recipes and make sure that this is safe for you to try.

The book is very specific to a physical and emotional condition. There are several recipes here because you might want to rotate and you may like one and not the other. There is also a variety of application. Some of us prefer to diffuse, some to make roller bottles, and others to create sprays.

I hope you enjoy this compilation, feel free to use the notes section and jot down your fave blends. There is a wonderful world of EO blending - this is just the beginning.

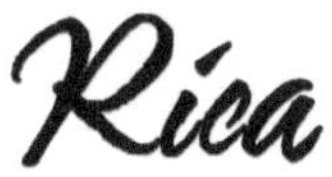

Table of Contents

Essential Oils For Pain and Inflammation

Bergamot: Bergamot is helpful when it comes to reducing and relieving inflammations. It has a natural antibiotic component that helps reduce and eliminate infections that results to inflammation. It also has this antispasmodic property that helps calm the muscles, increase blood flow and circulation to allow inflammation to decrease in a quicker healing time.

Camphor: Camphor has an analgesic and anti-inflammatory components that work together to ease the pain and inflammation felt in all parts of the body. With the help of its sedative properties, it allows the body to relax and calm down letting the bruises, muscle aches and/or pains and arthritis heal faster.

Clary Sage: Clary Sage is known for its anti-inflammatory and antispasmodic characteristic. The components it has helps reduce the pain felt upon the occurrence of inflammation that is cause by an infection or a bug bite. It also helps calm the body and mind allowing the person to relax and heal quickly.

Clove: Clove has an antiseptic property which is best in helping infected wounds throughout the body heal faster. It is commonly used to reduce pain and inflammation that is usually caused by headaches, swelling and joint muscle trauma. It also helps remove harmful toxins from that body that sometime can prevent proper healing to take place.

Eucalyptus: Eucalyptus has antibacterial properties which helps in cleaning and healing inflammation caused by infection, and easing the pain felt by this. Because of its decongestant properties, this is great in helping reduce inflammation that is caused by respiratory problems such as asthma.

Fennel: Fennel has an antiseptic component that helps promote healing of wounds or infection in any parts of the body, this also helps reduce inflammation in the affected area. Fennel's properties also serve as a stimulant that helps promote blood flow and circulation throughout the body to let the healing process be faster. It also has a component that helps remove harmful toxins from the body that might be slowing down the healing process.

Frankincense: Frankincense is great in reducing inflammations. It has sedative properties that relieves pain associated with the inflammation experienced, the said property also helps calm, relax, and allowing the person to rest in order to promote healing. The antiseptic properties it has also helps heal and prevent further infection that can sometimes cause inflammation to worsen.

German Chamomile: German Chamomile has great anti-inflammatory components that is perfect for relieving symptoms of inflammation. It also helps reduce the pain that is associated with inflammation in a way that it soothes and calm the body allowing the anti-inflammatory properties do its work. German Chamomile is also high in antioxidants which helps get rid of the bad toxins in our body.

Ginger: Ginger has anti-inflammatory properties that works together with the anti-nausea properties it contains to help reduce the pain and inflammation that can occur in the stomach. It also helps reduce inflammation that are caused by headaches, colds, muscle strains and arthritis.

Helichrysum: Helichrysum is best used in relieving pain and inflammation caused by arthritis. The properties it has helps remove toxins that may contribute to the inflammation in our body thus can promote healing to the body.

Juniper: Juniper helps remove toxins that can cause the inflammation experienced. The properties it has help increase blood flow and circulation allowing the white blood cells to get to the affected area to gain faster healing. Juniper also help relax injured muscles in order to prevent further inflammation in the body.

Lavender: Lavender has a therapeutic property that is a great help in relieving inflammation. It helps the body to relax in order to reduce pain and inflammation on affected areas. It also has the properties that helps calm skin disorders such as psoriasis or eczema.

Patchouli: Patchouli helps reduce Inflammation in the body by treating the areas that triggers inflammation. Its antiseptic property helps reduces fever and teats depression that can cause inflammation. The sedative it has helps relax the body to rest so that the healing process is faster.

Peppermint: Peppermint has properties that helps relieve inflammation. It has pain reducing properties that helps reduce stiffness. It also reduce redness and cools the affected area.

Rose: Rose is great in helping relieve inflammation that is associated with many health problems. It helps reduce inflammation that is associated with depression, stress, fevers and muscle spasm. It helps reduce the pain felt because of the inflammation.

Rosemary: Rosemary is great for helping reduce blood inflammation at the same time increases blood flow and circulation to help with the healing process. It has anti-inflammatory properties that helps treat muscle pain as well as rheumatism.

Sandalwood: Sandalwood has been used for years in helping to reduce and relieve inflammation. It has antiseptic components that help reduce and eliminate infections that causes inflammation. It helps soothes the affected area of the inflammation providing the body relief from the pain of the inflammation.

Sweet Marjoram: Sweet marjoram has properties that make it a beneficial essential oil to use when helping to reduce inflammation. It helps reduce pain associated with inflammation caused by muscle injury and arthritis. It also has sedative properties that are important in the healing process our body does.

Thyme: Thyme has anti-inflammatory and antispasmodic properties which are important in helping to reduce and relieve inflammation in the body. It helps increase blood flow and circulation to promote healing and removal of harmful toxins in the body. It is very helpful in relieving arthritis symptoms such as inflammation and pain.

Vetiver: Vetiver helps calm and soothe the affected areas of inflammation. It has antiseptic properties that helps reduce further infection. It also helps promote tissue growth which can be really helpful during the healing process.

Wintergreen: Wintergreen also helps reduce pain that is commonly associated with inflammation due to headaches. It has the same component as aspirins have which makes it an effective pain reliever. It also has the components needed to reduce the inflammation caused by an infection..

Yarrow: Yarrow helps in blood flow and circulation that relieves inflammation that is associated with arthritis. It helps reduce inflammation in areas like the digestive and respiratory system. It also helps promote healing and in the removal of harmful toxins in our body which slow

down the healing process

The Blending Process

These EOs are categorized by aromas, and EOs from the same group usually blend fantastically together.

- Floral – Lavender, Geranium, Jasmine
- Woodsy – Pine, Cedarwood
- Earthy – Vetiver, Patchouli
- Herbaceous – Marjoram, Rosemary, Basil
- Minty – Peppermint, Spearmint, Wintergreen
- Medicinal – Eucalyptus, Frankincense, Melaleuca
- Spicy – Pepper, Clove, Cinnamon
- Oriental – Ginger, Patchouli
- Citrus – Wild Orange, Lemon, Lime

Select oils that will give you with the health benefits you are looking to remedy. For increased energy choose: Grapefruit, Lemon, Orange, or Citrus. For Calming and Relaxation choose: Lavender, Cedarwood, or Chamomile. You are encouraged to experiment and play with your oils to see which blends work for you.

TIPS:

- Combine Floral EOs with Woodsy, Spicy and Citrus aromas
- Minty EOs with Woodsy, Earthy, Herbaceous and Citrus aromas
- Earthy EOs with Woodsy and Minty aromas
- Citrus EOs with Floral, Woodsy, Minty, Spicy and Oriental aromas

Diffuse

Diffusing Essential Oils is the safest method to enjoy Essential Oils without the risk of an allergic reaction.

Diffusing Essential Oils
Some Tidbits You Need To Know

Our sense of smell is one of our most powerful senses, and as you have noticed in your own experience that some scents affect your more positively in your minds than others. The body contains over 1,000 receptors for smell—way more receptors than for any of our other senses.

Diffusion Essential Oils means the process vaporizes oils into air by releasing tiny amounts into the air. Inhalation is totally safe and is super low risk. Chances of any EO rising to dangerous levels while diffusion is slim to none.

Diffusing Essential Oils around newborns, babies, young children, pregnant or nursing women, and pets should be done with caution. Read up on safety.

It is advisable that Diffusing Essential Oils for only about 15-30 minutes at a time to be most effective. NEVER leave your diffuser on overnight. Make sure your diffuser is filled with the right amount of water and you understand the operating directions.

While diffusing essential oils, be sure that your space has great ventilation. Crack a window open if the scent become to strong.

Never add Carrier Oils to your diffuser. This may cause your diffuser to malfunction. Clean your diffuser at least 3 times a week with warm water and natural soap to ensure the diffuser is well maintained and bacteria and mold does not accumulate.

Diffusing Essential Oils
Basic Guidelines

Just a few things you need to know and prepare before getting started Diffusing Essential Oils.

Things you need:
Ultrasonic Oil Diffuser
Essential Oils
Water

Just follow the number of drops in the recipe, drop on to an oil diffuser and fill the rest with water.

All diffusers are different and will have its own water minimum and maximum level. Read the diffuser instruction before use.

Ideally, it is best to diffuse for 15-30 minutes and turn off the diffuser. The effect should be good for at least 2-3 hours. Turn your diffuser back on after 3 hours to reinforce oil diffusing effects.

It is not advisable to use EO in humidifiers.

These are not made to release EOS

Diffuser Recipes

Here's a thought for you:

You may be wondering how aroma can simply eliminate physical pain. There's a simple answer to this : Pain whether coming from physical or emotion share the same space in our brains. Since emotions are closely connected to the sensory centers of the brain, what we feel emotionally can manifest, through pain we feel physically

So for here are a few recipes that can help you manage your emotions so it reduces the negative effects it may manifest in the physical body.

5 drops Bergamot
3 drops Frankincense
4 drops Rose
***

5 drops Bergamot
3 drops Frankincense
4 drops Rose
2 drops Peppermint
2 drops Myrrh
***

9 Drops Rosemary
5 Drops Melaleuca
4 Drops Geranium
3 Drops Peppermint
2 Drops Eucalyptus
2 Drops Lavender"
***

2 Drops Marjoram
2 Drops Thyme
2 Drops Rosemary
2 Drops Peppermint
2 Drops Lavender
***

1-2 Drops Marjoram
1-2 Drops Thyme
1-2 Drops Rosemary
1-2 Drops Peppermint
1-2 Drops Lavender
***

2 Drops Sweet Marjoram
2 Drops Thyme
2 Drops Rosemary
2 Drops Peppermint
2 Drops Lavender
***

2 Drops Peppermint
2 Drops Lavender
1 Drop Eucalyptus
1 Drop Rosemary
***

4 Drops Lavender
4 Drops Peppermint
2 Drops Frankincense
2 Drops Basil
***

2 Drops Lavender
2 Drops Wild Orange
1 Drop Geranium
1 Drop Clary Sage
***

3 Drops Peppermint
2 Drops Eucalyptus
1 Drops Myrrh
***

3 Drops Frankincense
3 Drops Lavender
3 Drops Bergamot
***

2 Drops Rosemary
2 Drops Peppermint
2 Drops Lavender
***

5 Drops Clove
2 Drops Frankincense
2 Drops Lemon
***

5 Drops Lavender
3 Drops Lemongrass
2 Drops Peppermint
***

3 Drops Coriander
3 Drops Peppermint
3 Drops Rosemary
***

3 Drops Lavender
2 Drops Cedarwood
2 Drops Vetiver
***

3 Drops Spearmint
2 Drops Tangerine
***

2 Drops Lavender
2 Drops Wild Orange
2 Drops Wintergreen
2 Drops White Fir
***

4 Drops Grapefruit
3 Drops Fennel
***

2 Drops Wild Orange
2 Drops Bergamot
2 Drops Cypress
2 Drops Frankincense
***

3 Drops Lavender
3 Drops Bergamot
***

3 Drops Peppermint
3 Drops Lemon
2 Drops Orange

Bonus Diffuser Recipes

Sinus Pressure Release

3 drops Peppermint
3 drops Lemon
3 drops Eucalyptus

Sinus Clear

2 drops Oregano
2 drops Tea Tree
2 drops Peppermint
2 drops Lavender
2 drops Lemon

Germ Killah

3 drops Tea Tree
2 drops Lavender
2 drops Peppermint

Sinus Head Tension Tamer

4 drops Lavender
4 drops Peppermint
2 drops Frankincense
2 drops Basil

Just Breathe Right

3 drops Eucalyptus
3 drops Peppermint
3 drops Rosemary

Tension Release Vapor

3 drops Frankincense
3 drops Myrrh
3 drops Cedarwood
(optional - to lighten the aroma a bit)
3-5 drops Orange
(optional - to add a sweet, fruity aroma to the blend)

Easy Peasy Stress Away

3-4 drops Lavender
2 drops Frankincense
2 drops Orange

Roll

Essential Oil Roller Bottles is the easiest method to enjoy Essential Oils Anywhere and Whenever.

Blending Essential Oils in a Roller Bottle
Some Tidbits You Need To Know

Essential Oils are usually super concentrated and too hard to measure how much to actually put straight from the bottle.

Roller bottles are a way that you are able to create blends ready to use with the right dilution. It allows your EO to last longer.

It also makes it easier to apply exactly where you want to target without getting it all over the place.

It is handy and easy to carry in your purse, ready to use at any time you want to.

I like to apply EOs at the bottom of the feet for many reasons. Our feet have bigger pores than any other skin in our bodies. this means that they are able to suck in the therapeutic compounds in our blend into the bloodstream faster that any other parts of the body. Imagine comparing a normal straw to an oversized straw and how much more you can suck in with the latter. This is how the soles of our feet is compared to the rest of the skin in our bodies.

The skin on our feet is also less sensitive and is designed to withstand some abuse. The risk of having an irritation from EOS is less likely to happen when applied on the feet.

The feet don't have the glands that act as a barrier. Sebaceous glands are glands in our skin that produces an oily substance called Sebum, for the purpose of lubricating and waterproofing the skin. Since this is oil and if you put oil on top of oil, it can act as a barrier or it may slow down penetration.

The feet and palms of our hands are the only skin that don't have these, so it is ideal to apply Essential Oils to the feet for maximum penetration.

Now, it would be hard to apply oils directly and very mess, right? Roller bottles make it super easy and convenient to roll the EOs at the bottom of our feet.

Carrier Oils Info

Carrier oils are vegetable-based oils with their own healing properties that dilute essential oils used to help carry the EOs into the skin.

Essential oils are highly concentrated and could evaporate very quickly. The carrier oil is mixed with the essential oil so it could penetrate the skin before it actually evaporates. Although EOs are oils, it is actually not that oily. When mixed with a carrier oil, it allows you to have more of the essential oil into your skin without wasting EOS to evaporate, making the healing properties of the EO strong and more effective.

There are also Essential oils that are too strong to apply directly to the skin and may cause damage, so it is important to dilute them with a carrier oil.

Never add Carrier Oils to your diffuser. This may cause your diffuser to malfunction. Clean your diffuser at least 3 times a week with warm water and natural soap to ensure the diffuser is well maintained and bacteria and mold does not accumulate.

Carrier Oils

There are a lot of different carrier oils that you can use with EOs to dilute them in a roller bottle.

To name a few :

Almond Oil - moisturizing and stays liquid at room temperature. Do not use if you are allergic to nuts.

Apricot Kernel Oil - moisturizing and suitable for sensitive skin or kids. It is super gentle on the skin.

Avocado Oil - moisturizing and suitable for sensitive and damaged skin. Perfect for skin problems.Can be mixed with other carrier oils

Castor Oil - with antibacterial, antiviral and antifungal properties, use topically to eliminate pain and relieve skin irritation.

Coconut Oil - its antibacterial, antiviral and antifungal properties it is the best and most versatile for skin care. The skin absorbs this very quickly. It solidifies in room temp and may still have a slight coconut oil aroma in it - but you can get a fractionated coconut oil to eliminate the 2 challenges above.

Grapeseed Oil - not just for cooking but also great for topical application on the skin.

Jojoba Oil - one of my faves for skin care blends. This oil is the closest to our natural oil our skin produces to it is absorbed easily without being oily. Also amazing for massage oil blends.

Olive Oil - this is the oil for herb type oils. mostly used for cooking but can also be applied to the skin but would need to be blended with a carrier oil that is mild and absorb well with the skin.

Rosehip Seed Oil - super good for deep moisturizing or skin irritations. This oil has a high content of antioxidants and helps remedy dry, scarred and wounded skin.

Recommended Roller Bottle Dilution Guide

RECOMMENDED ROLL-ON BOTTLE DILUTION AMOUNTS

5 ml (1/6 oz.) Roll-on Bottle = ~100 drops (1tsp.)
10 ml (1/3 oz.) Roll-on Bottle = ~200 drops (2 tsp.)
30 ml. (1 oz.) Roll-on Bottle = ~600 drops (6 tsp.)

Roll-on Size	5 ml	10 ml	30 ml	Add EO drops to roll-on, then fill with carrier oil.	
Essential Oil Drops	1	2	6	1%	Dilution Percentage
	2	4	12	2%	
	3	6	18	3%	
	5	10	30	5%	
	10	20	60	10%	
	20	40	120	20%	
	25	50	150	25%	
	50	100	300	50%	

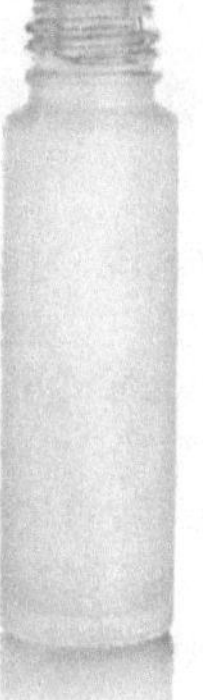
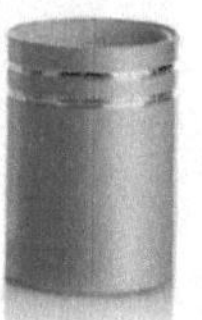

General Guidelines:
Birth to 12 months = .3-.5% dilution
1-5 years = 1.5-3% dilution
6-11 years = 1.5-5% dilution
12-17 years = 1.5-20% dilution
18 years and older = 1.5% dilution-Neat (no dilution)
Elderly or Sensitive Skin = 1-3% dilution
Daily Use = 2-5% dilution
Short Term Use = 10-25% dilution
Local Skin or Systemic Issues = 50% dilution-Neat

These are general guidelines suggestions--not absolute rules--based on traditional aromatheraphy practice.
(Kurt Schnaubelt PhD, Valerie Worwood, Robert Tisserand)

Dilution Basics:

How much you dilute your EO depends on different factors such as weight, sensitivity, health conditions, EOs that are blended in or how long that blend has been used for. There is never an absolute dilution rule, it is you who knows about your level and tolerance. I feel that it is best to start with a higher dilution percentage and increase EO drops over time.

To make sure your EO is safe, make sure that the oils you use are therapeutic grade and do your research on the source and extraction methods used to produce the oils.

Roller Bottle Blending Order

I normally just start with dropping the drops of oils into the **10mL roller bottle**, then adding the carrier oil up until the shoulder of the bottle. Capping the bottle off with the roller and the bottle cap. Instead of shaking the bottle, i like to roll the bottle between my palms first for a minute or 2 for blending, then finishing it off with a few shakes.

NOTE: All recipes in this book is for a 10mL Roller Bottle. If you have a bigger or smaller roller bottle, adjust the number of EO drops based on the size of your bottle.

Roller Bottle Recipes

5 drops of Lavender
5 drops of Lemongrass
5 drops of Frankincense

****

5 drops of Lavender
5 drops of Lemon
3 drops of Peppermint
3 drops of Eucalyptus.

****

5 drops of Lavender
2 drops of Frankincense
2 drops of Ylang Ylang
2 drops of Grapefruit.

****

6 drops of Lavender
3 drops of Frankincense
3 drops of Lemon.

****

5 drops of Peppermint
4 drops of Lavender
3 drops of Eucalyptus.

****

5 drops of Peppermint
5 drops of Orange
3 drops of Grapefruit.

****

4 drops of Frankincense
4 drops of Ylang Ylang
4 drops of sandalwood
4 drops of patchouli.

****

3 drops of Black Pepper
3 drops of Oregano
3 drops of Peppermint
3 drops of orange
3 drops of cedarwood.

****

5 drops of Lavender
5 drops of Frankincense
3 drops of Vetiver
3 drops of Ylang Ylang

****

4 drops of Peppermint
4 drops of Marjoram
4 drops of Helichrysum
4 drops of Wintergreen

****

5 drops Rosemary
3 drops Juniper Berry
4 drops Lavender

****

4 drops Peppermint
3 drops Oregano
2 drops Cedarwood
2 drops Lavender

****

3 drops Oregano
4 drops Peppermint
2 drops Cedarwood
2 drops Lavender

****

7 drops Lavender
6 drops Eucalyptus radiata
5 drops Juniper

****

5 drops Copaiba
3 drops Sweet marjoram
3 drops Basil
3 drops Frankincense

Bonus Recipes

Inflammation Massage Oil Favorite

60mL Jojoba Oil (cold pressed)
8 drops Lavender
8 drops Peppermint
15 drops Frankincense

Inflammation Massage Oil Secret

14 drops Frankincense
10 drops Sweet Orange
8 drops Turmeric
30mL Sweet Almond Oil

Inflammation Bath Soak Blend

10 drops Frankincense
5 drops Lavender
5 drops Bergamot
1 cup Full-Cream/ Full-Fat Milk

Inflammation Bath Salt Blend

1 cup Epsom Salt
¼ cup Dead Sea Salt
¼ cup Baking Soda
8-10 drops Essential Oils
(use any ingredient above or single oils)

Inhale

Essential Oil Inhalers are the most convenient way to enjoy Essential Oils Anywhere and Whenever.

Essential Oil Inhalers give you quick and easy access to the vast therapeutic benefits of essential oils.

Blending Essential Oils in an Inhaler
Some Tidbits You Need To Know

EO Inhalers or aroma sticks are compact tubes, with a cotton wick inside and a protective cover, to lock the aroma within.

Your preferred blend of essential oils is absorbed by the cotton wick, and safely enclosed in a tube that that fits inside of the cover. The cover is easily removed for access to the tube to breathe in the aroma. Usually lasts about 3 months, depending on the oil blend used.

I absolutely love these because they encourage me to take a moment during super stressful moments, and just breathe.

It is in times of stress when our breathing patterns often change and taking deep breaths promote a feeling of calm and inner peace. Breath work combined with visualization plus a relaxing inhaler, can offer relief to symptoms of stress and help your body to come back to the state of homeostasis.

Aroma Sticks can be carried in your tiny purse, even compact enough to fit in your pocket. You can enjoy your favorite EOs anywhere and you can use them with discretion.

I love diffusing, and do all the time but not everyone in my space may enjoy the scents I enjoy or they may not benefit from the therapeutic benefits of the EOs I am diffusing - so the inhaler is one way to not only enjoy my choice of blends but to keep in personal not affecting everyone else around me.

Inhalers not only benefits me but also keep those around me safe in case the oils I want to blend may pose a risk to those around me who may have health issue not advised to be exposed to my choice EOs/

When making Aroma Sticks, You may use your chosen EOs at 100% Concentration.

Inhaler Basic Guidelines

Breathe in slow and deep to absorb the EO molecules directly into your olfactory system.

Inhalers are super easy to use. You just remove the cap and inhale from the inhaler tube, count 1 to 5 slowly as you inhale. The EO molecules get drawn into our bloodstream through our nasal cavity and gets delivered throughout our entire body.

Simple to use, easy to cary, portable and compact. You never have to be without your favorite blends, ever.

Inhaler Blending Basics

Inhalers are super easy and simple to make.

All you need is an inhaler set which consist of the following:

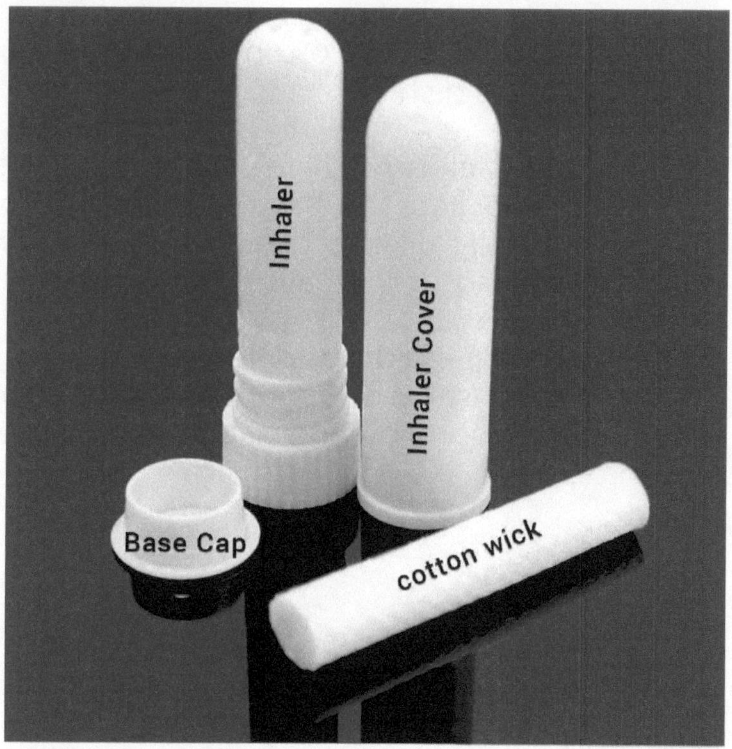

Inhaler, Inhaler Cover, Base Cap and Cotton Wick.

You will need your Essential Oils.

I like to use a pipette for precision and a small petri dish so I can see the oil.

Blending is super easy, just combine the drops and swirl it around in the petri dish and when you are satisfied you can go ahead and drop the cotton wick to absorb all the oil in the dish.

Once the wick is ready you can drop it in the inhaler and cap the bottom with the Base Cap. I usually like to secure the cover with the inhaler so I don't have to do it later.

I usually us 15-20 drops of EO total in a recipe and it can last up to 3 months. Some recipes will need more but on average it is in this range.

Inhaler Recipes

6 drops of Balance
4 drops of Eucalyptus
3 drops of Lemon
2 drops of Lime

****

5 drops of Frankincense
6 drops of Lavender
4 drops of Wild Orange

****

5 drops RC
2 drops Peppermint
2 drops Frankincense

****

3 drops of Lavender
3 drops of Lemon
3 drops of Melrose
3 drops of Eucalyptus
3 drops of Radiata
3 drops of RC
3 drops of Peppermint
3 drops of Copaiba

****

1 drop of Lemon
2 drops of Eucalyptus Radiata
3 drops of Rosemary
2 drops of Peppermint

****

4 drops of Peppermint
4 drops of Eucalyptus
2 drops of Lavender
2 drops of Lemon
2 drops of Rosemary

****

4 drops of Eucalyptus
4 drops of Siberian Fir
4 drops of Peppermint

****

5 drops of Wild Orange
5 drops of Bergamot
5 drops of Sandalwood
5 drops of Ylang Ylang

****

8 drops of Roman Chamomile
8 drops of Lavender
6 drops of Marjoram
1 drop of Vetiver

****

6 drops of Peppermint
3 drops of Frankincense
3 drops of Lavender
3 drops of Chamomile

****

3 drops of Oregano
3 drops of Tea Tree
3 drops of Lemon
3 drops of Frankincense
3 drops of Cinnamon Leaf

****

6 drops of Spruce
4 drops of Eucalyptus
3 drops of Lemon
2 drops of Lime

****

5 drops of Frankincense
6 drops of Lavender
4 drops of Wild Orange

****

6 drops of Eucalyptus
3 drops of Roman Chamomile
6 drops of Frankincense

****

4 drops of Thieves
2 drops of Frankincense

2 drops of Lemon

Book Ordering

To order your copy / copies of

please visit:
OilNaturalEmpress.com

You can also check out other titles available.

Bulk Pricing and
Affiliate Programs Available